10 Hacks To Destroy Fat

Destiny S. Harris

. . .

. . .

1st Free Gift!

Giving Rocks.

I give away free books daily.

Get your free books today.

Here's how

Step 1: Visit amazon.com/author/destinyharris

Step 2: Filter books by "Price: Low to High"

Step 3: Download available free books

. . .

Table of Contents

. . .

Chapter 1: Sever "Sugar"

You might be someone who says they don't like sugar. Well, I'm here to be the bearer of bad news. The truth is you probably **love** sugar.

I know several people who are overweight or on the thicker side who <u>say</u> they don't like sugar; their bodies tell a different story.

Sugar doesn't only include desserts. It includes your favorite Starbucks latte, your favorite beer, that bottle of wine you drink on the weekends, and simple carbs (e.g., chips, fries, crackers, bread, pasta, etc.). Everything is sugar.

Food companies want to put sugar in foods because that's how they keep you addicted and buying them; it's why I'll probably never give up Doritos.

You can splurge your way to the ideal goal you set for your body weight, but why potentially slow down the process?

If you're overweight, you've had enough treats. The proof is in the pudding. It's not a bad idea to take a break sometimes from what we enjoy. I promise you won't die.

Instead of splurging on your way to the finish line, sever the cord with sugar; this will expedite the process, eliminate (or decrease) cravings, and keep your body and mind focused.

One of the most challenging habits to implement is experiencing a cheat (or treat) day and getting back on track.

After you experience all of your favorite sugary things, your body wants more.

Sever the cord to prevent this while you're on your fitness journey.

This approach is similar to a person who finds out they have lung cancer. Many people continue smoking cigarettes.

Why exacerbate the issue?

Quit the thing or habit that got you here in the first place.

. . .

Chapter 2: Quit The Vine & Barley

Alcohol is an international favorite. According to the World Health Organization, over 3 billion people consume alcohol.

People love their drinks. I'm not for or against alcohol, but if you're trying to lose weight and live a healthier lifestyle, it wouldn't be the worst idea in the world to quit alcohol.

Whether your drink of choice is liquor, wine, beer, etc., the extra calories, the extra sugar, the effects on your liver, and the decrease in energy are all possible effects if you partake.

I'm going to use bodybuilders as an example.

One of the last things they should be consuming when preparing for a show is alcohol **throughout** their prep. It will only slow them down, take a heavy toll on their liver, and offset their gains.

When you have a health goal, you want to eliminate anything that can deflate your energy, vitality, and progress.

Quit the vine and barley.

. . .

Chapter 3: Fasted Cardio Only

A woman waved me to come over to her in the gym the other day and asked how to eradicate her hard, large gut. She was doing cardio on a stationary bike when she asked me this question.

I asked her a few questions:

1. What are you doing after you get off this bike?

The best thing you can do to eradicate extra fat is to perform resistance or weight training.

After completing her stationary bike cardio session, she told me she was heading home.

What she needed to do instead of the stationary bike was hit the weights.

2. Are you doing this cardio fasted, or did you already eat?

When you do cardio <u>after</u> eating, **you're burning off the meal.**

When you do cardio <u>before</u> eating, **you're burning off fat.**

Which do you think will get you results **<u>faster</u>**?

Option 2.

Of course, cardio can help, but weight training and fasted cardio will get you there faster.

There is no reason to make things more challenging and longer on yourself.

When is the best time to conduct fasted cardio?

First thing in the morning.

The woman ate a meal before she hopped on the stationary bike. Though she was working out her heart (good), she wasn't working off the gut (the goal).

3. How often do you do weights?

If you're not lifting weights, you're not maximizing your results.

I've been lifting weights since I was 11. I officially joined the gym when I was 14.

Weightlifting has kept my metabolism fast over the years. I can't become overweight because I've maintained an active lifestyle for so long.

When I take sabbaticals from the gym, I never overeat or consume too much of anything to the point my physique deviates.

Prioritize weightlifting over cardio.

Prioritize fasted cardio over cardio.

4. Are you lifting heavy?

Every time you hit the weights, you should safely increase the amount of weight you lift.

The more muscle you have, the less opportunity for fat and the quicker your metabolism.

The more weight you can lift, the more muscle

you tend to have.

. . .

Chapter 4: Prioritize Resistance Training

As mentioned in Chapter 3, you must prioritize weightlifting (aka resistance training).

Cardio will get you a healthy heart (and weightlifting can, too, when you do more circuit-oriented training), but weight training will get you a healthier, stronger, and more attractive physique.

I say resistance training because it is all-encompassing.

For example, mountain climbers and bikers are both resistance trainers.

The key is muscle.

You want to be adding and maintaining muscle constantly. The more muscle you have, the less fat your body tends to hold.

Furthermore, the more muscle you have, the more fat your body will naturally burn due to faster metabolism.

Practicing resistance training for decades has allowed me to coast with my fitness regimen.

I can go days or weeks without being in the gym and still maintain a slim and toned physique.

If I eat heavy or not so great one day or one or two weeks, there won't be any significant consequences.

Weightlifting grants you flexibility. If you're overweight, you probably like to eat, binge, or eat certain types of food.

Cool. I'm not judging you. I love food, too.

The best part of weightlifting is that it allows you to get away with eating how and what you want more often.

I was chatting with a 50-something-year-old in New York. He looks phenomenal. What is his secret? **Weightlifting**.

He started weightlifting in middle or high school and is the only one who looks two decades younger out of his friend group.

The rest of his friends look to be one to two decades older than him -- even though they're all the same age.

Want to eat more? Lift more weights.

. . .

Chapter 5: Quit Carbs

Quitting carbs is not necessary, but I noticed that my body was flatter, more toned, and any excess was obliterated. The results were tremendous. If you ever want to expedite the lean-out process, quit carbs.

What did I replace carbs with? Well, protein and fats.

My meals looked like this:

Example 1

Scallops, avocado, raw spinach

Example 2

Protein shake, boiled eggs, raw spinach

Example 3

Ground turkey, avocado, salsa, raw spinach

Example 4

Eggs, apple sausage, protein shake, raw spinach

What can I say? I like spinach like Popeye.

. . .

Chapter 6: Drink More Water

We often think we're hungry, but we're actually dehydrated.

Before you eat a meal, drink 1-2 glasses of water.

After you finish a meal, drink 1-2 glasses of water.

Right when you wake up, drink 1-2 glasses of water.

Right before you go to bed, drink 1-2 glasses of water.

Trust me, the more water you drink (as long as it's not too much relative to your body weight), the better.

<u>Drinking water also provides the following benefits:</u>

1. Keeps you hydrated

2. Decreases brain fog

3. Improves your mood

4. Increases your energy

5. Decreases sugar cravings

6. Keeps your metabolism moving

7. Keeps you full -- preventing overeating

The list continues to grow. There are countless benefits of drinking water.

How to Drink More Water

Keep water with you at all times. Keep it at your desk. Keep it by your bed. Keep it in your bag. Keep it in your car. Keep it next to you while you're at work if you work outside.

We tend to consume things that are within our line of sight.

Drink up.

. . .

Chapter 7: Keep It Out Of Sight

I like Oreos, Doritos, and ice cream. But I don't keep them within my line of sight. In fact, they're at the bottom of my pantry in a box.

The only time I consume them is when I **REALLY** want them. Otherwise, I'm not eating them.

Too many people have pantries and refrigerators full of their favorite delights. The more of your favorite treats you have easily accessible, the more you tend to eat.

Unless you have a high degree of discipline, what's at home gets consumed.

If you want to eat less ice cream, don't bring it home; if you do, get a small container instead of a large one.

Make the things you want hard to access.

I put the stuff I like all the way downstairs, at the bottom of the pantry, in a box. If I really want to eat it, I must put some effort in.

Besides a few snacks, my fridge and pantry are full of clean eats—everything else I have to put in effort to attain, which is how I prefer it.

The more stuff you have available and accessible, the more frequently you will give in to your temptations, which can all take you off track from your health and fitness goals.

Make the things you want to eat hard to obtain.

. . .

Chapter 8: The Order You Eat

My sister is a genius. While traveling abroad, she introduced me to the technicalities of the proper eating order.

The funny thing about this is I was subconsciously eating in the proper order but didn't realize it consciously. I ate in proper order because I hated how I felt when I didn't.

Ever feel like a piece of shit after eating pancakes for breakfast?

Or maybe you decide to have that sugary latte first thing in the morning; it's for energy, yet you experience a minor or major crash at some point.

The Proper Way To Eat

1. Start with the greens.

2. Integrate the proteins.

3. Integrate the fats.

4. Integrate the carbs.

5. If there's room for dessert, go for it.

Whether I'm eating breakfast or dinner, I start with the greens. My green of choice is raw spinach. It's easy to consume, fast, and easy. But

I love other greens, too, and variety is always best.

Always do your greens and proteins before you introduce the carbs. This helps avoid glucose spikes (which are not beneficial for your health) and reduces the likelihood of overeating.

When you eat your food in proper order, you likely have less room for carbs and dessert, which isn't the worst problem in the world.

...

Chapter 9: Sustainability

Ever notice when you cut out something completely (e.g., carbs, sugar, alcohol, eating out), sometimes you integrate back into your life with a vengeance?

Everything I recommend in this book is optional.

All of the strategies can work, but how you want to lose weight is up to you.

Choosing diet pills, surgery, or eliminating the things you love most might seem to be the best option that offers quick wins initially, **but is it sustainable?**

You probably don't want to get under a knife and potentially risk your life every time you gain too much weight (well, some of you might, but this is an unnecessary risk).

You probably don't want to subject yourself to endless types of pills. A lot of pills have many underlying effects we're not aware of.

Why not choose a more sustainable option?

I enjoy lifting weights and walking. I used to run seven miles a day and do multiple hours of spin class, but this is no longer sustainable, nor do I enjoy it anymore.

Biking outside is fun to me, though, which is sustainable. Sometimes, I don't feel like lifting weights, so I keep the workout short and sweet. I'm still getting the benefits, and it's sustainable because I don't hate it.

People frequently lose weight and then put it back on because the methods they leveraged to lose weight weren't sustainable.

You must find a method that makes it easy to maintain over long periods.

What does a sustainably healthy lifestyle look like for you?

It might mean going out dancing every night of the weekend, doing a fasted walk every morning, doing short mini at-home workouts throughout the day, or lifting weights intensively for 15-30 minutes each day.

It might mean eating out three times a week, eating out once a week, or adding a small dessert to each meal.

It might mean giving up certain foods altogether.

In high school, I gave up soda.

*Some things are worth giving up because they do
not add value to your health.*

I never smoked cigarettes. I don't believe in
heavy pharmaceutical use. And I aim to work out
3-6 times a week. Some weeks are more active
than others, but one thing I always do is walk.

I never start my day with coffee. I allow myself
to indulge in cravings, and when they've
subsided, I get back on track.

If they haven't subsided, I sometimes allow
myself to indulge longer or force myself to get
back on track to remind myself that I'm in
control, not food.

Discipline is a critical trait; without it, you will never reach your goals. Always remind yourself of your goal and what you're willing to sacrifice for it.

Pain (or discomfort) is a necessary part of the process of becoming a healthier version of yourself.

What does a sustainable regimen look like for you?

. . .

Chapter 10: Measure

<u>What gets measured improves.</u>

I've never been a scale person. I don't even own one. In fact, I've never owned one or bought one before. I usually weigh myself 1-3 times a year.

I don't care about my weight as long as I look and feel great.

However, if you're overweight or obese, measuring your progress is productive. What doesn't get measured *may* improve, but likely at a slower rate.

If you're lifting weights, you might not always notice a drop, **or you might.** But if you weigh 300 pounds and want to get down to 200 pounds, you should measure your progress by hopping on that scale.

When you measure, you are holding yourself accountable.

Don't measure daily.
Instead, measure weekly.

Write down the number and focus on your actions to reach your goal the following week.

Never obsess over numbers.

Instead, focus on living a sustainably healthy

lifestyle.   54

. . .

Thank You For Reading

Thank you for reading this book.

Stay blessed, lucky, favored, aware, joyous, and committed to bettering yourself.

. . .

The End.

. . .

About Destiny S. Harris

Destiny S. Harris' goal is to positively inspire, cultivate, elevate, and educate the minds of individuals across the globe through her writing.

Creating (whether books, courses, articles, poetry, or music) has always been Destiny's thing, not to mention health & fitness and all things entrepreneurial. Destiny published her first book, "Beauty Secrets for Girls," at age 11 and her second book, "Don't Wait Until It's Too Late," at age 12.

Destiny obtained three degrees in Psychology, Political Science, & Cultural Studies. She also started her own music teaching business at the age of 14, which she led for over ten years. In addition, she has been teaching academic, career, and personal development topics to thousands of students and readers since 2004.

Outside of writing, Destiny loves and enjoys a few other things: reading, weightlifting, traveling, football, dogs, food, classic movies, mountain and ocean views, sleeping, plants, and nature.

Check out her work, leave a review, share your thoughts with your friends and family, and be a part of a movement: helping people learn and grow through means of self-education (books).

<u>**Complete the Steps To Get Free eBooks:**</u>

Step 1: Go to amazon.com/author/destinyharris

Step 2: Filter books by "Price: Low to High"

Step 3: Download available free books

. . .

Connect W/ Destiny S. Harris

Please reach out and stay in touch. Destiny S. Harris enjoys chatting with readers.

Start a conversation today @ destinyh.com

. . .

Free Gifts!

Access courses & free eBooks at the link below:

destinyh.com

. . .